Prologue

As we age, nearly all of us develop chronic conditions which make living a little less pleasurable. We experience levels of discomfort in our muscles, joints, digestive tract, urinary tract and organ systems which, while not life threatening, take some of the joy out of living. The author, quite by accident, stumbled on MSM as a nutritional supplement which has measurably improved the quality of his life. He gives credit to the devoted practitioners of veterinary medicine for pointing him in the right direction. And to his dedicated pharmacy instructors at the University of Michigan in the 1950's for giving him the analytical skills necessary to identify and interpret, with minimal bias, improvement in the human condition in response to treatment with MSM.

MSM

A Pharmacist's Perspective

by **Ron Jones, Rph,** Retired

Content

How it Started
The Broccoli Diet
Veterinary MSM
My Disease
My I.C. Diagnosis

Additional Anecdotal Observations
MSM and my PSA
My Auto Immune Connection
Geographic Tongue
Knee Pain
Back Pain
Exercise and Urethritis
Cataracts
The Eyes Have it.
Colon Polyps
Human Allergies

How it all Started

It started in my early 40's with symptoms of prostatitis. I experienced a burning sensation every time I urinated, and the symptoms lingered for a significant period of time. My urologist took urine samples, then prescribed antibiotics. They had zero effect on ameliorating my symptoms. The urologist eventually settled on periodic prostate massages as a temporary fix. Then, when I was 49, I had a urinary tract bleed which was correctly diagnosed as bladder cancer, and surgically removed the next week. The urologist said pathology reports identified the lesion as LOW grade, and he gave me a 95% chance of it never recurring. It never has, although a U of M urologist stated that once a person gets bladder cancer, they are always at risk of recurrence.

We never identified the cause of my bladder cancer, but as a pharmacist, I frequently (daily) compounded chemotherapeutic agents (cancer drugs) without benefit of a special I.V. Hood to protect me from the carcinogenic substances. Our hospital was going broke, and couldn't afford the special equipment. But our cancer patients needed the drugs. Cancer drugs which suppress the disease process in small doses, can cause cancer in higher concentrations over time. I can't blame the urethritis on the exposure to chemotherapeutics, because I had the symptoms years before that exposure took place.

The Broccoli Diet

About the same time, my chronic non-bacterial cystitis, urethritis spread to my testicles. Periodic ultrasounds proved negative, so I've just lived with that as well. My urologist's response to this symptom was: "Well, some guys get that" ! At one point, about 15 years ago, I couldn't go anywhere without a doughnut seat cushion. Even in Church, I took my little black doughnut. Finally, in sheer frustration, I discovered the Broccoli diet. Lyda bought a vegetable steamer, and I ate steamed broccoli three times daily until I gagged. Wow, looking back, that was pure torture. But over time, it seemed to help. I surmise it was the sulfur content that was doing the job.

Discovering Veterinary MSM

About the same time, our golden retriever, Topbrass Kelly, was showing signs of hip discomfort. I found a product on Foster and Smith that looked promising, so we gave it a try.

The product brochure stated that the active ingredient, in addition to glucosamine, was MSM. The product information stated that MSM was slow to achieve therapeutic levels, and that the dog owner should give the product for at least 6-8 weeks before expecting to see results. As it turned out, the MSM product proved to be VERY effective, but in fact, took nearly two months to achieve the desired therapeutic response.

Coincidentally, I was having significant bilateral shoulder pain (due to the adverse effects of fluoroquinolone antibiotic) on the tendons which attach my rotator cuff muscles, so decided to give MSM a try to relieve the symptoms. My family doctor recommended Ibuprofen, but that drug killed my 96 year old grandmother before we knew much about its proclivity to cause gastric hemorrhage. A few doses of the drug gave me heart burn...and I stopped. Now we know that long term use can also predispose users to heart attacks. Two reasons not to use it. So off I went to the local pharmacy in search of MSM. Well, two months later, my shoulder pain was significantly reduced...but more dramatically, my UTI symptoms had abated. What is going on, here ? Why am I getting up fewer times during the night and having significantly less burning

when I Pee ? Could it be the MSM ? At the
time, I was taking a moderate dose, which is half
of the maximum dose suggested by the
manufacturer. Can't remember the generic brand
I was using at the time, but it was sold by a local
big box store.

My Disease

Let me say up front that I have never been
definitively diagnosed with prostatitis and
interstitial cystitis. Both are presumptive
diagnosis, based on my symptoms. The
symptoms first appeared when I was in my 40's,
and initially were treated with antibiotics
(Declomycin), presuming that the cause of the
burning and inflammation in my urinary tract
was bacterial. That type of treatment would
continue through several urologists...culminating
in three months of therapy with fluoroquinolone
antibiotics. The antibiotic therapy had ZERO
effect on my symptoms, but the extended Cipro
& Levaquin therapy did result in the eventual
loss of my rotator cuff muscles in my shoulder.
It is now common knowledge that
fluoroquinolone antibiotics can attack vulnerable
tendons...most notably, Achilles tendons. It just
happened that my Rotator Cuff musculature was
the most vulnerable. As a younger man, I played

basketball, tennis, golf, hunted with shotguns and was an Alpine Ski Patroller. Except for shooting light recoil shotguns, I've lost the ability to participate in any physical activity which requires sound rotator cuff musculature. But that is another story. Suffice it to say, I have mixed emotions about the medical practice of urology, except to say it saved my life in correctly diagnosing and surgically eliminating bladder cancer in 1985. I've been getting annual cystoscopic examinations for the past 33 years, without recurrence of the disease. But the non-bacterial urethritis, which has migrated to my testicles, has persisted to this day... And MSM has been my salvation in that regard.

My I.C. Diagnosis

I was originally told that I probably had a male form of interstitial cystitis, although my University of Michigan Urologist questioned that diagnosis because I lack the one symptom which she said most IC patients experience. Discomfort radiating from the bladder in the lower abdomen. So I can't say definitively that I have the same condition many female patients complain of. And because the breakdown of the top layer of my digestive/urinary track mucosa is so extensive, I can't be sure I have the same disease as many of you have. All I can say is, there seems to be NO evidence that I've had an infection over the past 40 years, and the symptoms are controlled when I don't loose my mind and stop taking MSM.

Other Anecdotal Observations

MSM and my PSA

Last year my urologist told me that my PSA, after decades of moving up very slowly to the low 3's, had jumped up into the 4+ range. He said my overly large prostate was still soft, so because of my age and urinary tract inflammation, it was possible that I was not developing prostate cancer. But to be sure, we should repeat the test in 30 days. It wasn't until I got home that the light came on. Two months before I had, again, stopped my MSM to see if it was doing any good. Could that have been at the root of my elevated PSA ? So I want back on MSM. And I waited <u>two</u> months before I repeated the PSA. Well, you have already guessed the answer. The repeat test was back in the low 3+ range. My urologist asked me if I would send him more information on using MSM for chronic,idiopathic, non-bacterial prostatitis and interstitial cystitis.

My Autoimmune Connection

In 1996, on the 4th of July, I developed a painful blotch on my tongue. Some time later, I was diagnosed by my EENT specialist with geographic tongue (autoimmune disorder), but at the time it was just one more insult to my digestive mucosa. I was already experiencing heartburn whenever I ate acid, fat or highly seasoned food, so this seemed to be just an extension of that process. It was at this point in my life that my diet started to change significantly. No more citrus fruit, or any product preserved with citric acid. And no more chocolate. I soon learned that ANY seasoning was bad for my tongue, my heartburn or my cystitis. Lyda started cooking basic, non fat, unseasoned foods. And did I say that Alcohol was a no no ? Guaranteed irritation from any alcohol product. For the past decade, meals have consisted of a basic meat sans seasoning, a boiled potato, and unseasoned vegetable. I do use salt for seasoning with no change in symptoms. I don't take vitamins, except for 125 mg of Vitamin C every other day to ward off Scurvy. The other drugs I take are One Gram of Glucosamine daily, Metamucil three times daily and one baby aspirin daily. When I go on a Glucosamine drug holiday, I can perceive no difference in my symptoms.

Yes, I'm a pharmacist who takes NO prescription drugs..save for an antibiotic to treat rare sinus infections.

Geographic Tongue

I talked briefly about geographic tongue. When the condition was first diagnosed, I had all of the mercury based amalgams drilled out of my teeth (with protective dams to prevent the material from being swallowed). That didn't help. I continued to have painful, denuded areas on my tongue for years, and couldn't drink a pop, eat a piece of fruit or eat candy with citric acid content. Anything acid set off the tongue. My local dentist suggested Biotene tooth paste and rinse. That helped. Not a cure, but it made the condition tolerable if I avoided any food product that was acid. But over an extended period of time, my tongue is nearly normal. I suspect that my geographic tongue & frequent heartburn when I eat fruit or fatty foods is related. In fact, I suspect that the highly sensitive mucosa all the way from my tongue to my urinary tract is an autoimmune disease. Bad Genes ! Sorry Mom and Dad...not your fault.

Knee Pain

Three years ago I developed intense, bilateral knee pain during my daily walk in the forest trails next door with my Golden Retrievers. Temperatures were single digits, and I wasn't sure I could make it back out of the woods after the intense knee pain hit me. A local orthopedic specialist took X-Rays, then sent me to physical therapy. The therapy actually made the condition worse. After a month, I quit. Over time, the symptoms abated somewhat, but going for our daily morning walks was torture. I eventually discovered on my own that exercise biking gave me moderate relief. The symptoms persisted for over a year, but gradually returned to tolerable levels of discomfort. As I write this, it suddenly occurred to me that the knee pain is almost gone. Not completely, but MUCH more tolerable than it was even 1 year ago. My orthopedic guy and my family physician both say that my problem is arthritis...but I think their diagnosis is formulaic. I don't have arthritis in other joints. But I have had tendon problems for decades.   I had to quit playing tennis because of chronic tennis elbow... and the pain feels identical to the PAINFUL TENDONS I had when I was more athletic.

Back Pain

In the mid 90's, Lyda and I took our Golden Retriever hunting dog to visit our daughter in up state Wisconsin. Her husband invited us to come in October and hunt Grouse. Birds were plentiful, and Kelly was showing signs of being a reliable bird dog on local pheasants. Dave piled us into his classic Jeep, and we headed down logging roads looking for good grouse cover. Kelly was petrified of riding in the back of the open Jeep, and insisted on riding in my lap. If you ever have an opportunity to ride over rough logging roads with a 65 lb dog in your lap...Don't ! When we returned after the hunt, I took a hot shower and lay down on the couch. I wasn't able to stand up straight again for three days. Every bit of connective tissue in my back had been stretched to the point of injury...and I was in serious pain. The pain lingered for at least two years. I went to an Orthopod, and the exercises he prescribed made it worse. I had to roll out of bed in the morning, and had to stop my routine exercise running program. I tried using Capsaicin topically, but it was ineffective. Exercise always made it worse, and even rubbing the small of my back set me up for extended pain. I missed a pheasant hunt in South Dakota the next fall..much to the disgust of my pheasant hunting partner.   And from that point on, any time I rode in a car for over an hour, it set me up for prolonged back pain for the next few days. Occasionally, I would have to roll out of bed during the middle of the night and crawl on my hands and knees to the bath room.

Now, it is quite possible that, over the next 2 decades, the back finally healed. The dramatic improvement I've seen in those symptoms occurred most notably after I started taking MSM. But the improvement was far from instant.

Exercise and Urethritis

Before MSM, I couldn't treadmill, or engage in any exercise which involved rapid or rigorous movement of my legs. The rapid movement of tissue in the groin area set me up for extended discomfort. I could go for walks with our Goldens in the woods, but I couldn't run, jog, or ride an exercise bike. That changed over time as I continued to take MSM. Now I can ride my exercise bike for 20-30 minutes without any meaningful effect on my urinary tract symptoms.

Cataracts

Many of us who spend time in the sun will develop eye cataracts as we age. I always had a sense that I was predisposed, genetically, to that significant health issue. I've spent a lot of time outdoors when I was younger, playing tennis and golf in the spring and summer, hunting with my dogs in the fall, and spending a lot of time on Michigan's Alpine ski slopes (in the glare of sun off of the snow) in the winter. I vividly recall a communication with my father when he was almost exactly my age (82), informing me that he was going to have cataract surgery. Dad had retired to Florida, and lived adjacent to a fairway on the golf course he played regularly. He and his golfing partner were very close to the same age, and both had developed cataracts to the point where they could no longer follow the golf ball in flight, and couldn't find their balls on the fairway to take their next shot. It got so bad they had to have golfers on an adjoining fairway help them find their balls. The cataract surgery was a great success, but it is not something you want to undertake if you can avoid it. Lyda had cataract surgery recently, and complications made the recovery an unpleasant experience.

The Eyes Have it !

As an avid outdoor sportsman and upland bird hunter, one of my favorite clay target games is the original game of skeet. We call it Vintage Skeet. Without boring you with the details of the original rules, "Shooting Around the Clock" as it was called in 1935, is significantly more challenging than modern skeet rules. It requires the rhythm, timing and dexterity of a golf swing with the precision eye sight of a marksman. Rotator Cuff physical therapy (and MSM?) allowed me to retain my dexterity into my 80's, but my genetic predisposition for cataracts had me worried. A local Ophthalmologist warned me in 2001 that I was about a year away from requiring cataract surgery.

Well, that was over 18 years ago. Can I give credit to MSM for stabilizing the deterioration of my eye sight due to cataracts ? Absolutely no way to know. But given the fact that I managed another rare 25 straight at the game of Vintage Skeet just two weeks ago, I'd have to give credit to something other than my father's GENETICS !

Colon Polyps

Nearly all of us have a routine colonoscopy periodically to assure that we are not developing colon polyps. Certain types can evolve into colon cancer. About the time we moved to Midland, the local Gastroenterologist reported that I had developed a type of colon polyp which could develop into a cancer. He removed the polyps, and said I needed to repeat my colonoscopy every 3 instead of every 6 years. More polyps developed three years later. They were again removed, and I was told to repeat the colon exam in another three years. About that time, I started taking MSM and, it's important to note, began taking a baby aspirin daily based on recommendations from a cardiologist. At that time, aspirin was indicated for any patient with a family history of heart attacks. The medical community also observed that patients on a daily dose of aspirin MAY be less subject to the development of colon polyps. Fast forward to last year, I've been free of colon polyps for 12 years, and my gastroenterologist proclaimed that I no longer required a routine Colon exam. There is no way to know whether the MSM or the Aspirin, or both, eliminated the formation of polyps in my colon. But I sure like not doing colonoscopies any more !

Human Allergies

I've been an allergy sufferer for 75 years. I started with asthma and hay fever. As I matured into adulthood, the asthma resolved, but the hay fever tormented me for decades. Fall ragweed was brutal on my eyes and nose. Two decades ago now, I took allergy shots for three years, and the fall allergies abated...but, they were replaced with spring allergies. The spring allergies start in April, and seem to go on well into the summer. The Hay fever resolved before I started MSM, and thus far, MSM seems to have minimal or no effect on my spring allergies. Allegra is effective for the spring allergy symptoms, but if I don't take it...my sense is that the MSM is having no effect. I understand that many people give MSM credit for reducing their allergy symptoms, so I'm going to relate to you my observations with one of our Golden Retrievers.

The Canine Patient

The beauty of canine patients is their honesty. They don't lie. You can't ask them how they feel. When Abby feels and moves better, you can clearly see it in her eyes and her drive. When her allergies are kicking up, she chews her feet. And if her G.I. Spasms return, the swallowing symptoms are obvious. Psychosomatic disease symptoms and a placebo drug response are not a factor in documenting my observations. It makes therapy evaluation more objective.

Canine allergies

Two years ago, Abby developed classic canine allergy symptoms. One morning we came home from our run in the forest, and she started licking her paw. Close inspection revealed inflammation between the pads. Douxo Calm Mousse gave her some relief, but the symptoms continued into the spring. Soon, all four feet were effected, and she had to wear double cotton sox on all four feet to keep her from licking her feet raw. Antihistamines proved to be totally ineffective. But the vet had an answer. A veterinary drug company had developed a monoclonal antibody (MAB) drug to counter canine allergies. It worked. But based on the manufacturers clinical studies, the $100.00 shot only lasts for an average of two months. Each shot, as it turned out, was effective for close to 60 days. Then the paw allergy returned. At this point I started MSM. I told the vet I was giving Abby one gram a day, and he thought that was too much. He advised 500mg daily for a 65 lb dog. But I've continued the one gram dose. After the first two months of MSM, her time to relapse has averaged close to 4 months.

It's important to note that she has shown ZERO signs of ANY adverse effects from MSM. Stools are perfectly normal. Since putting her on MSM, we've seen a noticeable improvement in the appearance of her coat.

Canine Esophageal Spasm and MSM

When our female Golden Retriever was two, she developed a gastric condition that resulted in frequent bouts of repetitive swallowing. That, in turn, usually lead to vomiting and diarrhea. We would stop her dog food, put her on a rice and boiled chicken diet for three days, and the condition usually resolved. Michigan State Vet school said their gastroscopy revealed NO pathology. Just keep her on a diet of predigested dog food (Ultamino), give her NO treats, and give her omeprazole 20mg daily. That was a significant improvement, but whenever we tried to taper her off of the Prilosec, or reduce the dose, the symptoms came rushing back. If she got one "tiny" lick of her birthday cake icing, it set her up for extended repetitive swallowing jags the next day. That happened on more than one occasion. Then we put her on MSM for her allergies.   After two months, her repetitive swallowing condition appeared to improve. To test my hypothesis, I tapered her off of the Prilosec for a month and she remained nearly symptom free. That's the first time in three years that she has been able to go without the drug. And her energy levels dramatically improved. Before the introduction of MSM and before discontinuing omeprazole, she would spend most of her afternoons hiding under the bed. After discontinuing the Prilosec, she displayed energy levels nearly identical to young Jak. She still had an occasional bout of repetitive swallowing, but it usually resolved quickly and did not resulted in vomiting or diarrhea. Again. This is anecdotal..so don't take it to the bank. I just throw it out there to confirm that there is a lot of *circumstantial* evidence to suggest that there may be broad spectrum application for MSM in seemingly unrelated medical conditions. The drug/nutrient appears to facilitate reversal of insults to tissue, irrespective of the cause.

Canine Seizures

Eldorado's Jak O' Hearts is a 2.5 year old field bred Golden Retriever. He's a close relative to Abby. On Feb 1st of 2017 he experienced a tonic-clonic seizure with a recovery lasting about 40 minutes. The first 10-15 min. were violent. He experienced additional seizures about every 4 months. We started him on MSM 1 gram almost exactly a year later. He's experienced subsequent seizures at about the same interval over the next year, but it is worth noting that they were drug induced. He experienced a seizure following doses of Benadryl, Nexguard, and Flagyl. What we've noticed is that the tonic-clonic portion of the seizures is significantly shorter. Seizure episodes still last about 40 minutes, but the violent segment of the seizures are much shorter, and significantly less violent. Coincidence? No way to know.

My Thoughts on MSM

Is MSM an Analgesic ?

Many authors refer to the analgesic effects of MSM. As a pharmacist, when I say analgesic, I'm referring to drugs which are capable of ameliorate acute pain with a single dose. Got a headache ? Take a Tylenol and most people feel some relief in about half an hour. Knee pain? Take Ibuprofen and you should be feeling less pain within days. Analgesics and non-steroidal anti inflammatory drugs, within the context in which they are normally prescribed, don't require months of therapy to achieve some measure of effectiveness. When we refer to MSM as an analgesic, I worry that patients will get the idea that a single dose will relieve pain, the same as aspirin and hydrocodone. I like to think of MSM as a REALLY SLOW ACTING anti-inflammatory. It does not appear that MSM works to block nerve pathways, preventing nerve innervation to relay pain signals to the brain. And in fact, it may not be a drug at all, Looks to me like it is an essential nutrient the body needs to repair tissue damage. When the tissue damage is repaired, the pain and burning abate. But that is PURE conjecture on my part. You are free to disagree.

The Effects of Caffeine

Caffeine is a common chemical in our daily diet. Many of us consume beverages which contain caffeine. You'll be delighted to hear that my experience with caffeine has been extremely positive. My urine flow is improved, and the urinary tract inflammation is minimal when I consume moderately caffeinated black coffee. Others might not share my experience. Each individual is different. But I drink 4-5 cups of moderately caffeinated black coffee daily throughout the day.

Effective Dose

So Ron. What dose should I take for my symptoms ? Sadly, in this litigious society, I not only can't tell you what dose to take...I can't tell you to take MSM at all. Every human is different. A drug or nutritional supplement which is beneficial to one person may not be beneficial to another. And a dose which is effective for one, may not be for a second. And most important, even though many report limited to no side effects with MSM, you may encounter a serious, even life threatening adverse reaction.

My hunting partner started taking MSM last year, and while he was taking it had episodes of angioedema. Did the MSM cause it? He doesn't know. He still takes MSM, and the facial swelling is gone. But I certainly would not want to advise you to take MSM and have a serious, life threatening event. Evaluate my experiences as they relate to your condition...then consult with a trusted medical professional who knows your medical history for advice on this one. There may well be other drug/nutritional products better suited to your condition.

MSM..the mystery nutrient

So Ron, if MSM is so great, why aren't drug manufacturers and physicians touting the virtues of MSM ? That is a really great question, and the answer appears to be rooted in our free enterprise system. Let me start to answer that by defending free trade and the lack of government control over our economy. If there is anything that governments do well, I haven't identified it. Everything they touch turns to...well, you know what I'm about to say. Now I'm not saying that there is NO place for government in the development and distribution of pharmaceuticals, because left to their own devices without some guide lines, free markets can go astray. Our markets are driven by the almighty dollar, and that is a strong incentive. Companies like Microsoft and Apple went from garage operations in their infancy to world domination because of profit incentives. If governments were controlling every aspect of the pharmaceutical industry...including profits, we'd still be treating syphilis with mercury. It's the profits which can result from the development of a superior product that motivates pharmaceutical companies to produce the next greatest drug.

But to answer your question, there is NO profit incentive in funding an expensive drug evaluation for a compound which...(A) has never been proven to cure anything and (B) is cheaper than dirt. And in fact, you can probably identify a few molecules of MSM by analyzing the dirt in your back yard. It's a common chemical in our environment and in our food. Biologists tell us the organic chemical starts out as a by product of decaying plankton in the bottom of the ocean...morphs through a couple of chemical stages until, in a gaseous form, evaporates into the clouds. Then it cycles back down in the next cloud burst to provide nutrition for plants and animals. Our ancestors ate the plants and animals, which resulted in MSM becoming an integral and essential part of our biology.

Unfortunately, today's food preparation practices is said by some to remove or destroy much of the naturally occurring MSM in our food.

Medical community in the Dark

Over time, I began to wonder about the long term use of MSM ? Internet searches said that the product was extremely safe. In researching the product, I discovered that it was related to DMSO, a pharmaceutical urologists instill into the bladder of people afflicted with interstitial cystitis. But my urologist assured me DMSO was not a cure..just temporary relief of symptoms. I had already had enough annual cystoscopies to make sure my bladder CA hadn't returned, so more insults to my ultra sensitive urethra was not something I was willing to do. And when I asked my urologist, my family physician and his nursing professional what they thought of MSM ? Their eyes glazed over. And when I said, "MSM, that's methylsulfonylmethane" !! Their eyes crossed. They had no clue. My local veterinarian knows much more about MSM than many human health care professionals. So your doctor may have to do a little research on the product before he or she directs you to take it.

Is MSM a Cure?

My limited personal observations have suggested that MSM is Not a cure. Others who have used the drug claim that it is. It may depend upon the condition being treated. My conditions developed late in life, and my body may never be able to completely reverse tissue damage which has occurred over time. I'm still afflicted with the same irritating urinary tract conditions I've had since my 40's. That's about 4 decades, since I just turned 82. But what the drug has done is make living more enjoyable. I can't tell you how many times, before MSM, I irritated my dear wife by challenging her cooking. Any other woman would have thrown up her hands in total disgust. I'd accuse her of using garlic...or onions in a recipe. And caution her to never use tomato paste. She loves spaghetti, and she even tried making it without tomato paste. Good luck with that, ladies. Even soups and salad dressing contain more seasoning than I can tolerate. Getting up every night, every 45 minutes was not conducive to getting a good night's sleep. And then laying there in bed, staring at the ceiling until the burning stopped was not restful. That was then...and this is now. I still avoid pepperoni pizza, spaghetti and onions in my meat loaf, but at least I'm not making life miserable for Lyda. Yesterday we ate stuffed crust DiGiorno pizza, and today we ate vegetables seasoned with Blue Cheese Dressing. **I'm not cured**...but the improvement in the quality of life post MSM is enormous.

Side Effects

If your health care professional concludes that your medical condition could benefit from MSM, make sure you include a list of allergies. A number of drugs are sulfur based, including antimicrobials, anti-diabetics, diuretics and anticonvulsants.

The PLACEBO Effect

Let's stop and talk about the placebo effect for just a moment. In one of my first pharmacy classes, Dean Rowe told us about the psychological benefits of drug therapy. And how drug manufacturers frequently divided populations of study patients into a placebo group and a drug therapy group. The pharmacist dispensing the drug wasn't even told which patients were receiving the inert medication, and which were getting the drug being studied. Such studies are frequently referred to double blind, crossover studies, where the medical team evaluating the results doesn't know which patient received a therapeutic dose of medication, and which got a capsule packed with an inert sugar. That way, they could fairly compare the results of the two groups, and decide whether the drug had additional benefits beyond those benefits which can result from the power of positive thinking. It's common knowledge that if a patient perceives a positive benefit from the therapy when he or she starts taking a drug, they may well experience a positive outcome even if the drug was not responsible. The human mind is a very powerful thing, and we can't discount the psychological benefits which result from the patient truly believing that he or she will get better as a result of the therapy.

Placebo therapy for Erectile Dysfunction

I offer the following as a way of demonstrating the power of the mind. When I was a young pharmacist, fresh out of school, I puzzled when middle age male customers would come into the store and ask for Frank. Frank was a pharmacist, but also the owner of the drug store. One day I asked Frank what was going on. The customers, by word of mouth, discovered that Frank had a MAGIC medication in the back room of the pharmacy, which acted like Viagra. It was, they were told, a male aphrodisiac. Men who were impotent came to Frank for a small cardboard pill box of his special medication, and were so thrilled with their performance at home that they came back time after time for refills. One day I asked Frank what medication he was dispensing to the Gentlemen ? I wanted to know if he was breaking the law by dispensing a prescription drug illegally. He grinned ear to ear as he retrieved one bottle of blue and a second bottle of pink tablets from the back room. Both drug bottles were labeled *APC* tablets (Aspirin, Phenacetin and Caffeine). If the blue APC tablet quit working for a patient, Frank switched their medication and gave them a Pink APC tablet. Frequently, the Pink tablet would work when the Blue tablet failed. APC was a mild pain medication similar to Excedrin, with zero aphrodisiac properties. It was all in their heads...but it worked miracles.

So now you know what the Placebo effect is all about, and why it is nearly impossible to evaluate the true efficacy of a drug or nutritional product based on the experiences of a single patient. And why you should look with some skepticism on any finding, based on anecdotal evidence.

Psychosomatic Diseases

 I just went on one web site that stated that the average female patient ends up seeing 8-9 urologists before she finds one that takes her interstitial cystitis symptoms seriously, and explores options for relieving the symptoms. It is frequently also difficult for health care professionals to differentiate between symptoms which are the result of a true disease process, and which are psychosomatic. In my particular case, my urologist can't see any changes in my bladder mucosa, even with the intense burning I feel at times. But if my disease turns out to be psychosomatic, and the cure turns out to be the placebo (mind over matter) effect, does it really matter ? I firmly believe with all my heart (but not based on actual science) that my disease is real...and, that the symptomatic relief I experience from the MSM is also real.   There are just too many patients with similar symptoms, and too many patients who experience meaningful relief with MSM. But in the end, everyone should consider how powerful the human mind is...not only in imagining disease which displays no physical signs, but also in interpreting the curative nature of chemicals and

biologicals.
The Importance of Drug Holidays

As a pharmacist, I have an intense paranoia about long term side effects of drugs. When I was responsible for screening the drug therapy of patients in a long term care hospital, I frequently put patients on a drug holiday to see if they REALLY needed the drug. Naturally, I didn't do that for drugs which are life sustaining. But for drugs which ameliorate symptoms, it's very beneficial. If the patient's symptoms don't worsen while he or she is on a drug holiday, then most likely they don't need the drug. And it is not uncommon for many patients who are experiencing a worsening of their disease state are, in fact, suffering from an adverse drug event from one of their drugs...or from the combined effect of a drug cocktail. So I periodically put myself on a drug holiday from my MSM to see if it was actually producing a beneficial effect. However, I have to say that evaluating the benefits of MSM is difficult. The symptomatic benefits are slow to reverse, and symptoms can vary from day to day even during a period when I've been taking MSM for more than six weeks.

I know, what I don't Know !

So Ron. Given the placebo effect of drugs, and the possibility that your symptoms are psychosomatic, how can I be sure the drug will benefit me ? YOU CAN'T ! And that is why you should consult a health care professional to assist you in deciding whether or not to take MSM...to help you monitor any adverse effects, and help you decide whether you should continue to take the product.

What should be reassuring to you is that the experiences I have related, based on over a decade of treating an assortment of personal and canine ailments with MSM are based on a fundamentally sound scientific principal. **I know what I DON'T KNOW**. I understand the basics of a scientific study, and know that it takes a well controlled, double blind study comprising a significant population of patients over a long period of time to draw any meaningful conclusions about the therapeutic and adverse effects of a drug or dietary supplement. How many drugs have been withdrawn from the market after a decade of use in the general population because the researchers were not able to identify a life threatening adverse effect of the

drug in their clinical trials ? Many, Many, Many
! And even at that, most honest clinicians will
tell you that the findings based on small clinical
studies should be viewed with some skepticism.
Statistical sampling and evaluations based on that
science are not always easy to interpret.

So start by evaluating what I've said with a
measure of skepticism...but be reassured that my
experiences have been subjected to a great deal
of scrutiny and critical thinking to get to the
point where I am willing to share my experiences
with the general public. I want people to know
how MSM has significantly improved the quality
of my life.

Why I Trust my Judgment

So Ron. You already warned us that your
experience is anecdotal. Why would we trust
your judgment ? Well, that's because I have, on
multiple occasions, stopped taking the drug to
see what happens. And after about 6 weeks, my
symptoms come back WITH A VENGENCE !
Because of my age, I usually even forget that I
was taking the drug until suddenly, I realize that
it burns a lot every time I pee, I'm yelling at Lyda
for seasoning my food, and I'm getting up every
hour during the night to go to the bathroom. So I

go back on MSM...and yes, it takes six to eight weeks before I'm back to living and loving life again.

In Summary

It's important to reiterate. MSM is NOT an analgesic. At least, not in the way most health care professionals think of medications which relieve pain. Aspirin, Tylenol, Ibuprofen and controlled substance analgesics will relieve pain and discomfort after only a few doses. And in a relatively short period of time. By comparison, it usually takes four to six weeks minimum for MSM to achieve symptomatic relief. The changes are so subtle that many people may not perceive a measurable benefit during treatment. And in fact, only after the patient has gone on a drug holiday for another 4-6 weeks, will the true benefit be recognized.

Then why consider MSM for relief of Arthritis, Cystitis, and the vast assortment of related conditions for which others have claimed benefit from MSM treatment ?

Safety

If your condition will require long term treatment, perhaps for the rest of your life, consider the safety profile for optional therapies. Liver damage is said to be rare, but must be considered in long term use of acetaminophen (Tylenol). NSAID products, notably Advil, Motrin and related drugs, can erode the gastric mucosa over time. Hydrocodone and Oxycodone opioids can lead to drug addiction over time. And if you review the extensive list of side effects from corticosteroids, it will make you think twice about long term therapy.

By comparison, MSM appears to be relatively free from side effects. However, there is no guarantee that MSM is appropriate for your condition. And despite the safety profile of MSM, at some point in treatment you may experience an adverse reaction to the sulfur containing compound. Only your personal physician can determination whether MSM is an appropriate alternative to conventional drug therapy...and monitor your progress accordingly.

Before you purchase MSM

Let me just use Webster's definition of a word which is not frequently discussed in conjunction of Generic drugs. **Bioavailability:** *the degree*

*and rate at which a substance (such as a drug)
is absorbed into a living system or is made
available at the site of physiological activity.*
As a Pharmacist, I've always been acutely aware
that not all formulations of a pharmaceutical, or
in our case, a nutritional substance, are the same.
The purity of the chemical compound in question
is essential if you don't want to introduce
impurities into your body. And the formulation
of the solid or liquid dosage form is important if
you want your body to be able to utilize the
drug/nutrient to maximum efficacy. Case in
point. Back in the 1980's I developed a drug
dosing program for our hospital which allowed
the Pharmacist to assist the physician in
determining the precise dose of a cardiac drug
which was used to alter the force and rate of
contraction of the heart for patients with
Congestive Heart Failure. The dosing program
was based on the pharmacokinetics of a heart
drug which was almost exclusively manufactured
by a leading pharmaceutical company. But about
that time, generic drug manufacturers were
gaining acceptance by the general public, and
since the patent had long expired on digoxin,
generic manufacturers began to market drugs
which were said to be "generic equivalents". As
it turns out, the generic products contained
exactly the same amount of digoxin as the brand

name product, but professional reviews were revealing that not all patients taking the generic were achieving therapeutic blood levels of the drug. We chose not to use generic products for our cardiac patients. Cutting to the chase...the generic products were not all formulated with the same care as the original brand named product, and the absorption, distribution and elimination characteristics of some of these products (there's that Pharmacokinetics word again) was not equal to that of the brand name product.

Since retiring from pharmacy, I assumed that our world of medicine had caught up with this phenomenon. But sadly, it had not. Lyda had been taking Coumadin for years as a result of heart valve surgery and occasional cardiac arrhythmia, but one day our new insurance carrier decided that they would only pay for the generic form of the drug. So our local pharmacist substituted a generic as required by the insurance company. Fortunately, Lyda was scheduled for her blood clotting test the next month, and her blood clotting times had moved out of the acceptable range. It's worth noting that her clotting times had been consistent, without exception, for years. Her Coumadin clinic clinician marvels at her 96% compliance...year after year. It was necessary to have her doctor write an "exception" report and send it to the insurer before she was permitted to go back on Coumadin, rather than a generic brand of warfarin. Her INR went back into the normal range the next month, and has stayed there for over a year.

My point is this. If you and your physician decide that MSM might improve the quality of your life, it is imperative that you choose your product carefully. Identify a company with an extended track record of producing quality products, and make sure the source of the MSM the drug manufacturer is using is as pure as humans can make it. Make sure the MSM is made in the U. S. of A.

Meet the Author

I was no different than any other kid growing up in rural Indiana in the 40's. I loved the outdoors. Roaming around adjacent corn fields with my Daisy Red Ryder BB gun, and shooting hoops in the back yard with my friends was what I lived for. Waterford was no different than thousands of other rural, mid-western K through 8 grades across America. Mr. Todd was the principal, and he also taught grades six, seven and eight in one room.   When he was instructing the sixth graders in reading, writing or 'rithmatic, it behooved the seventh and eighth graders to keep their heads in their books studying whatever subject constituted the current assignment. Mervin Chupp sat next to me, and he was one cool dude. Many of my classmates were Amish and Mennonite, and they grew up respecting American values. And in fact, I can honestly say that they were the epitome of American Values. We all horsed around at recess, but during class, Mr. Todd ruled with an iron fist. We knew that we were in Mr. Todd's class for one reason...and one reason only. To learn. And learn we did. I was awarded the Bausch and Lomb science award my Junior year at Owosso High (Michigan), and graduated in the top 5% of my class as a senior at Niles High.

Was I a child prodigy? Absolutely not. I just had parents and teachers who knew what was best for little Ronnie...and they made sure my education was well grounded in reading, writing, arithmetic and the sciences. Dad said I had the option of going to Notre Dame, where I could live at home and drive to class daily from Niles, or go to the University of Michigan and live on campus. Like most youngsters who are 18 years old, I wanted to to away to college, so I went to U of M. The curriculum choice was easy. All thorough high school, I enrolled in every science class available to me. But before that, I asked my parents for a Gilbert Chemistry and microscope set. The Chemistry set came in a suitcase filled with cylindrical wooden containers of chemicals. But the most impressive part of the chemistry set was the alcohol burner, test tubes, tongs and litmus papers. I learned more about chemistry with that Gilbert Chemistry set than most students learn in chemistry class.

Studying Science

So when I went to Michigan, it was logical that I would major in chemistry, with the goal of working for Dow Chemical company based in Midland, Michigan. But strange things happen to students along the way. By my sophomore year, I learned that students with a Bachelors degree in chemistry end up washing test tubes at Dow. I would have to extend my education another three years to earn a PhD in chemistry, and land a good job at Dow. Dad's resources were limited, so he suggested that I explore Pharmacy as an alternative. I could continue to pursue my passion in a science based curriculum, and get a degree that would land me a good paying job. At the time...and indeed until I retired from pharmacy 49 years later...there was no such thing as an unemployed pharmacist. So I walked into Dean Rowe's office in the University of Michigan Chemistry building and said: "Dean Rowe, I think I want to be a Pharmacist. The rest is history. I graduated with a 3.5 GPA in Pharmacy, and took a job as a community pharmacist in Saginaw. The father of one of my classmates owned a drug store, and he hired me straight out of school before I took the Michigan State Pharmacy Boards. From community pharmacy I moved on to Hospital pharmacy, because it allowed me to practice pharmacy in more fundamental ways. And in fact, before retirement, I developed a program for our hospital which applied pharmacokinetic principles to the renal excretion of drugs....allowing us to modify the dose of drugs which have a narrow margin of safety. Early experimentation with a Schering Pharmaceutical company computerized drug dosing program gave me the basics to apply the pharmacokinetic principles to the dosing of a broad spectrum of pharmaceuticals known to accumulate in the bodies of patients with compromised kidney function.

I've been fully retired for a decade, enjoying life to the fullest. But I have one nagging concern. Are there folks out there, like me, who would benefit from knowing about MSM ? If you are one of those with chronic ailments not responding to conventional therapy...ask your

Doctor about MSM.

Personal Health Notes